VEGETARIAN WEIGHT LOSS COOKBOOK

Dietary guidelines for vegetarians who want to lose weight

BETH LINTON

Table of Contents

CHAPTER ONE

Weight loss with a vegetarian diet

Dietary guidelines for vegetarians who want to lose weight

As long as you keep an eye on what you eat, you can lose a few pounds.

Vegetarianism is a lifestyle choice that can be made for a number of different reasons, including health and environmental reasons.

It has been shown that a high-fiber vegetarian diet reduces the risk of chronic diseases like heart disease and diabetes while also lowering calorie and saturated fat intake.

It can also help you avoid obesity, but it can be difficult to lose weight if you make a few mistakes.

Because of the high percentage of calories from carbs in vegetarian diets, dietitian Julia Zumpano, RD warns that losing weight can be difficult.

Losing weight on a vegetarian diet is possible, but it necessitates some effort.

explains what you might be doing incorrectly with your diet, as well as what you can do about it.

There are a few ways to go about a vegetarian diet, the most important of which is to avoid eating meat.

• Vegan. All animal products, including those found in meat and poultry as well as in eggs and dairy are strictly forbidden in vegan diets.

• Lacto-vegetarian. Meat, poultry, fish, and eggs are not allowed on this diet, but dairy products are.

• Lacto-ovo-vegetarian. Lacto-ovo-vegetarians don't consume animal products like meat, poultry, or fish, but they do consume dairy and eggs.

a vegetarian diet has a "restrictive nature," so it's important to make sure you're getting the nutrients that are more readily available in animal sources, such as calcium and B12.

How to lose weight if you're not seeing results

With regards to weight loss, those who eat a diet high in fat, moderate in protein, and low in starch and carbs are more likely to succeed.

For the most part, people on low-carb diets fared better than those on low-fat diets when it came to sustaining long-term weight loss. Because they consumed fewer carbohydrates, people on high-fat diets performed better than those on low-fat diets.

Many studies show that when you eat high-quality protein and fat, your lean body mass rises, while when you eat starch and sugar, it falls.

For those who are unable to shed the pounds on a vegetarian diet, here are some possible reasons why.

To many calories are being consumed.

When eaten in large quantities, legumes, nuts, and seeds, which are all sources of protein, are high in calories.

Vegans must consume larger quantities of these foods than meat to meet their protein needs, according to When it comes to protein, a 4-ounce piece of lean meat provides about 200 calories and 28 grams of protein. Cooked beans provide close to 400 calories to get the same amount of protein as that found in two cups of cooked beans."

A 1-ounce piece of lean meat provides 200 calories and the same protein content as a 1-

ounce serving of nuts, but the meat has only 55 calories.

Beans are a good source of protein and carbohydrate, so treat them as such when preparing a meal." advises against adding another carb, such as potatoes, pasta, or rice. When it comes to meeting your protein needs, you should eat a larger amount of beans.

If you're looking for a low-carb source of protein like tofu, seitan, tempeh, or a dairy product like Greek yogurt or cottage cheese, you can also opt for egg whites or egg white substitutes.

You're overdosing on refined carbohydrates.

The answer is yes. Carbohydrates are permitted in vegetarian diets. Nonetheless, many of us fall into the trap of eating an excessive amount of refined carbohydrates. There is no doubt that we're referring to pizza, pasta, and bread here.

CHAPTER TWO

Those options are low in fiber and can leave you with an unsatisfying sense of fullness. As a result, you're more likely to overindulge.

As an alternative, you should eat a diet rich in vegetables like sweet potatoes, butternut squash, oatmeal, and beans and lentils. These complex carbs, which are high in fiber, are better because they don't cause your blood sugar to rise as quickly.

As long as you keep your portion sizes in check and always include a protein source and plenty of vegetables when you eat pizza or pasta, it's fine to indulge once in a while," says "As an example, prepare a pasta primavera dish with a variety of vegetables and add chickpeas or lentils for protein. For dinner, I recommend a veggie pizza with fresh mozzarella and a green salad."

You're overindulging in calorie-heavy food.

Those on a vegetarian diet may find that foods high in fat such as nuts, butters and seeds as well as avocados and coconut can help them feel fuller longer. Nutritional and filling, these foods are worth a try. Despite the fact that a little goes a long way, it's easy to consume a lot of calories.

By tracking what you eat and drink, "you'll be able to identify foods that may be contributing to weight gain,"

To keep track of calories, you can use an app or write them down in a notebook.

Food that has been heavily processed is what you're consuming.

Eliminating meat from your diet increases your intake of processed foods.

While meat substitutes such as meatless burgers, sausages, veggie nuggets, and breaded patties are generally regarded as vegetarian alternatives to meat, they can contain a plethora of additives, sugars, salts, and preservatives.

"These foods are both convenient and delicious. It's important to keep track of your caloric intake to ensure that you don't overeat on these foods.

How to shed pounds on a vegetarian diet

So, how can you make positive changes to help you lose

weight? Listed below are a few ideas:

• Consume a lot of real food. You get the most original nutrients when you eat whole foods.

Consider cutting back on your intake of highly processed food. One to two times a week is all that's necessary.

Add some protein to your snacks. It's easy to forget about protein in snacks when you're eating your main meals. So, include seeds, beans, nuts, lentils, low-fat dairy, and eggs in your mid-afternoon pick-me-up.

• Include plenty of vegetables on your plate. Choose foods high in fiber, such as leafy greens, broccoli, cauliflower, and zucchini. You'll get a better sense of fullness and eat fewer calories as a result.

Vegetarianism is an excellent way to improve one's health. And it's not as difficult as you might think, thanks to a wide variety of cookbooks and recipes.

You may even be able to shed some pounds with some careful planning and tweaks. (Also, don't forget to get some exercise and sleep!)

Eating mostly plant-based foods has been shown to have numerous health benefits, even if it does lead to weight gain, says Zumpano. As the saying goes, "Eating a plant-based diet improves your health from the inside out."

Plan, shop, and prepare for your next trip to the store.

CHAPTER THREE

There is nothing more intimidating than making a major shift in your diet at first, but it does not have to be. To get through the first two weeks of a plant-based diet, follow these three simple steps:

1. Plan. Make a two-week meal plan. Even if they're not exactly the idealistic meals you see on Instagram, make them simple and give yourself some leeway.

2. Shop. After that, go shopping. A well-rounded plant-based pantry can be built even if you buy just a few items for the pantry once or twice per week. To help you get started, we've included a shopping list below.

3. Prep. Finally, if you find yourself lacking in motivation after work during the week, it's a good idea to do some pre-work ahead of time (prime hit-the-drive-thru time). Preparing all of your meals for the week at once can save you time and

effort (Sundays work well for many people).

Getting ready to go

Pre-plant-based days left you with a well-stocked kitchen? If you're done, you should be fine.

You'll need the following equipment if you're making the switch to a plant-based diet and cooking at home for the first time this year.

- a non-stick pan (s)

- pots with lids for cooking

chef's knife that is good

- a serrated bread knife is a must.

- blender

- strainer

measurement devices such as cup and spoon

- a variety of sized mixing bowls

- a sheet of aluminum foil

- Pan for bread or muffins

Mixing bowl with large spoon, large turner, and large spatula

- a can spout

Other appliances that may be useful in saving time and effort include food processors and air fryers as well as other types of rice cookers.

Simple changes

Since meat is obviously a no-no, what about all the other products made from animals that you consume on a regular basis?

Here are a few simple alternatives.

As an alternative to the following:

Try

a hen

An egg substitute made from flaxseed (1 tbsp flax meal and 2.5 tbsp water)

Scrambled tofu

the seeds of one type of plant, one type of plant milk, and a sweetener of your choice; refrigerate overnight before eating) or flavor-infused gelatin chia pudding

Ingredients: nutritional yeast, parmesan cheese

Plant milk, as opposed to cow's milk (soy, oat, flax, almond, coconut)

hummus made with mayonnaise (or vegan mayo)

In a nutshell, coconut butter

poultry/beef/veggie broth/stock (keep veggie scraps in a bag in your freezer to make it yourself)

Choosing a protein

A healthy plant-based diet necessitates an adequate supply of protein. (Fortunately, it's also incredibly simple.)

If you're not a vegan, you can get plant-based protein from nuts, seeds, soy products, beans, meat substitutes, and plant-based protein powders.

Plant proteins, on the other hand, don't supply enough of the essential amino acids to meet your dietary requirements, unlike animal proteins. There is no better way to ensure that you are getting enough of these vital AAs than by consuming a variety of plant-based proteins.

Your body will thank you for making sure to include a wide variety of foods rich in essential fatty acids.

Preparation of food for the week is easy.

Here's our foolproof method for meal prepping that works for everyone and any occasion (plant-based or not). If you like to batch cook on the weekends, this is a great way to plan your week's meals.

CHAPTER FOUR

To begin, choose a protein. Tofu is a good starting point for this discussion.

Add a grain of sand to the mix. Aside from rice, we could use barley, noodles, tortillas or anything else that comes to mind.

Finally, select a vegetable. Bok choy, here we come.

Stir-fried tofu, rice, and bok choy sound delicious, don't they? Add sesame seeds and green onions to the dish for garnish.

Hacks and cheats that we use the most frequently

Looking for a way to expedite the process? A few of our go-to tips for making a plant-based diet more manageable include:

Taco Bell, of course. Do not be offended. Even though the food is heavily processed, it is a viable option if none are available. You can find them almost anywhere, and they have a full Veggie Cravings menu that is certified by the American Vegetarian Association.

• Meal kits and delivery service. Consider a meal kit like Green Chef, Sunbasket, or Purple

Carrot if you have room in your budget (all of which send preportioned ingredients and recipes for you to cook your own plant forward meals). There are also fresh or frozen meal delivery services like Fresh N Lean (which offers vegan or low carb vegan meals) and Trifecta Nutrition if you're in a time crunch or just want an easy way to get a healthy lunch at work (which offers vegan or vegetarian plans).

• Preserved foods. Your fruit bowl would be free of mushy

brown bananas covered in fruit flies, and your crisper drawer would be free of liquefied bags of baby spinach. There's nothing wrong with having some frozen vegetables on hand in case you don't have time to prepare a lot of fresh vegetables. If you're looking to make some takeout-style rice, frozen pea and carrot bags are an excellent option, as well as frozen riced cauliflower, which can be used in soups and rice dishes alike.

Beans in a can. Similarly, canned beans are an excellent

option. Dry beans are less expensive, but they require more preparation time because they must be soaked, sorted, and cooked for longer. A few cans of different kinds of canned beans can come in handy when you're in a pinch and need a quick meal.

Grains that have been precooked. Precooked grains, such as rice and quinoa, are also a lifesaver for those who have a hectic schedule. However, the convenience of only needing to reheat the grains makes them worth the trade-off. Occasionally, you just want a delicious meal to be ready in no time.

Food that can be consumed quickly and is made from plants

Want something that'll be done quickly? You can count on us, veggie family. The following are a few quick, no-cooking-required meals that can be made in less than five minutes.

• PB&J. It's a time-honored film. Almond butter, local jam, and whole grain bread make it even better.

Avocado toast with chickpeas. With canned chickpeas, this is an easy, protein-packed dinner. Sprinkle with salt and pepper to taste and eat your way to millennial nirvana.

Beans and rice can be sped up by using shortcuts. All you need is canned beans, precooked rice, a few minutes in the microwave, and your favorite seasonings. Even if the beans and rice aren't the best you've ever had, they'll do for a quick hot meal.

• Salad made from whatever is in the fridge. Absolutely true to its word. Salad greens are a great base for a variety of leftover vegetables, nuts, seeds, plant-based cheese, chopped up veggie burger patties, or toasted chickpeas. Add your favorite plant-based dressing or simply drizzle with oil and vinegar.

In order to ensure that all of your nutritional needs are met on a plant-based diet, it is essential to supplement with a variety of vitamins and minerals. The following vitamins and minerals may be lacking in a plant-based diet:

fortified with B12

fats rich in EPA and DHA

- iron

- iodine

- zinc

- calcium

- D

- iron

- selenium

The majority of your nutritional needs should be met by a good multivitamin, but make sure it contains at least 100% of the Daily Value (DV) for vitamin B12 and an omega-3 vegetarian source. (Also, don't forget to eat seaweed! Iodine is a major component.)

Recipes for a plant-based diet

To get you started, here's a sample 14-day meal plan. 14 different breakfasts, noons, suppers, and desserts have been included for a total of 56 different meal and snack ideas. In any case, we strongly advise you to make changes so that you can make it your own!

For example, most people are fine with eating the same breakfast every day. So, for the first two weeks, stick with whatever breakfast sounds the best to you (or at least two or three). Even in the mornings, you'll be able to save some time. Even meals can be made this way if you're willing to give up a little variety for the sake of time and money savings.

Any of these meals can be served with a side salad or some steamed or sauteed vegetables that you have on hand.

THE END